Legal & Disclaimer

The information contained in this book is not designed to replace or take the place of any form of medication or professional medical advice. The information in this book has been provided for educational and entertainment purposes only.

The information contained in this book has been compiled from sources deemed reliable, and it is accurate to the best of the Author's knowledge. However, the Author cannot guarantee its accuracy and validity so cannot be held liable for any errors or omissions. Changes are periodically made to this book. You must consult your doctor or get professional medical advice before using any of the suggested remedies, techniques, or information in this book.

Upon using the information contained in this book, you agree to hold harmless the Author from and against any damages, costs and expenses, including any legal fees, potentially resulting from the application of any of the information provided by this guide. This disclaimer applies to any damages or injury caused by the use and application, whether directly or indirectly, of any advice or information presented, whether for breach of contract, tort, negligence, personal injury, criminal intent, or under any other cause of action.

You agree to accept all the risks of using the information presented inside this book. You need to consult a professional medical practitioner in order to ensure you are both able & healthy enough to participate in this program.

Contents

Introduction 5

Chapter 1 6

What is the keto diet? 6

Types of Keto Diet 6

Objectives of the Keto diet 7

Characteristics 8

Difference between a traditional diet and the ketogenic diet 8

Changes it produces in the metabolism 9

Chapter 2 10

How did Keto start? (Technology industry) 10

Why are dieticians against it? 11

Chapter 3 12

Side effects 12

How do you know if your body has entered a state of ketosis? 12

How to measure ketones in the blood? 13

Chapter 4 14

Benefits 14

Chapter 5 15

35 Nutritious and delicious recipes from Keto, easy to prepare with 5 ingredients and in only 15 minutes. 15

Soups 15

    1.   Corn and Tomato Soup 15

    2.   Sweet Corn Cream 16

    3.   Beetroot Cream 16

    4.   Light Artichoke Broth 17

    5.   Light Detox Broth 17

    6.   Fat-Remover Soup 18

    7.   Roast Vegetable Cream 18

    8.   Fresh Energetic Soup 19

    9.   Chicken Breast Consommé 19

    9.   Leek and Chicken Cream 20

Mains 21

1.   Chicken Breast in Oriental Sauce 21
2.   Mushroom with Pork Sautéed Au Gratin 21
3.   Lettuce Mix with Pork 22
4.   Pork with Julienne Mix & Mustard 22
5.   Dressed Salmon in Papillote 23
6.   Aromatized Chicken with Salad 23
7.   Beef Salad Roll 24
8.   Pork Sirloin with Coriander Sauce 24
9.   Aromatic Hake with Salad Mix 25
10. Cauliflower Veggie Pizza 26

Desserts 27

1.   Sweet Potato & Dry Fruits Bread 27
2.   Sweet Pineapple in Ron 27
3.   Cheese and Cream Keto Cake 28
4.   Delight of Cauliflower Rice and Coconut 29
5.   Sweet Keto Donuts 29
6.   Chocolate Fritters 30
7.   Dark Chocolate Stove Bread 31
8.   Avocado Keto Brownie 31
9.   Almond Fluffy Cupcake 32
10. Cappuccino Flavour Cupcake 33

Snack 34

1.   Cauliflower Croquettes 34
2.   Crispy Mozzarella Sticks 34
3.   Battered Vegetables 35
4.   Buffalo-Style Cauliflower Trees 35
5.   Battered Mango 36

Chapter 6 37

Food for consumption in the keto? 37

Drinks from the keto diet? 38

Foods to avoid or decrease in the keto diet 38

Chapter 7 39

Can I go on playing Keto forever? 39

How to avoid the rebound effect, after the diet? 39

The behavior of the kidneys with the Keto diet. 40

Chapter 8 41

Tips 41

Conclusion 42

Introduction

The ketogenic diet is a safe diet, which enjoys scientific support, and has been used as such since 1924. It has great prestige and is the most recommended worldwide, as a non-pharmacological treatment, to promote weight loss, prevent and improve health conditions.

The ketogenic diet has the same effects as fasting, after many scientific studies; it has been made more flexible, becoming today the best option to treat obesity, neurological pathologies, and in the prevention of modern diseases.

Carbohydrates and sugars produce a hormonal response that minimizes the production of ketone bodies, favoring the accumulation of fats in the body and leading to obesity. The ketogenic diet through the specific combination of macronutrients changes the functioning of the body's metabolism and stimulates the production of ketone bodies that support weight loss and improve health.

Keto Chef is a useful tool, with complete information about the ketogenic diet, its origin, its effects on the body, benefits to improve health conditions and to show off a stylish figure, as well as a lucid mind.

This issue contains 35 recipes of the keto diet, easy to prepare, with natural foods and preparation time of 15 minutes. Ideal for beginners, busy people with little time to prepare their food.

Keto Chef is an ideal guide for people who want to take care of their health and that of their family, as well as enjoy mental clarity and a healthy body, taking control of their life, in a fun way, saving time and money.

Chapter 1

What is the keto diet?

It is a diet high in fat, protein according to individual needs and very low in high fiber carbohydrates, perfectly combined with the purpose of producing ketone bodies.

The body is induced to the state of ketosis and in turn, the liver transforms the fat into ketones that naturally feed the muscles, brain and heart, without any problem.

It is a dietary intervention to raise the levels of ketone bodies in the blood, thanks to the combination of macronutrients, which changes the functioning of fat metabolism.

The ketogenic diet activates the body's natural defense system, forcing it to take the fats that are in reserve, to convert them into energy, so that the person can carry out his or her daily activities.

This mechanism helps to lose weight and to improve health conditions at a physical and mental level.

It is a diet that over the years, has acquired great prestige, positioning itself as one of the preferred by the fitness world, as a complementary dietary treatment and to maintain a healthy life. It is endorsed by the scientific community, for its proven effectiveness and the great benefits it brings to health.

From the point of view of ancestral feeding, people did not have easy access to carbohydrates and sugars; however, they enjoyed excellent health and longevity. This makes us think that we can live healthily with minimal amounts of these macronutrients in our diet.

According to expert statements, carbohydrates are non-essential nutrients and their theoretical value is zero.

Types of Keto Diet

There are many types of the keto diet, with particular characteristics, which have had to be modified and adapted to meet the individual needs of each individual.

The percentage of fat, carbohydrates and protein define the type of ketogenic diet, however, they all have a common goal which is the production of ketones. Each individual adopts the type of diet that is adapted to his or her needs and produces the results that he or she expects.

The procedures in which the ketogenic diet standard should be managed are

Carbohydrates 5-10%, fats 60% and proteins 30- 35%, according to the type of diet and individual needs of macronutrients.

Among the most common types of diets are:

1. Standard Keto

    The most recommended because it can be adapted to each specific case.

2. Keto Proteins

    Special for specific cases, which require higher protein content, such as sick people, pregnant women, sportsmen, etc.

3. Cyclical Keto

    It is a combined keto diet, which alternates 3 days of cyclic diet and 4 days of standard diet, or as the case may be.

    There are many versions of the keto diet, which have been modified and adapted according to the needs of particular macronutrients.

Objectives of the Keto diet

The main objectives of the keto diet are:

- Reduce bodyweight

- Improve health conditions

- Preventing diseases

- General welfare

Characteristics

-The main characteristic of this diet is that it suppresses or reduces to a minimum, the consumption of carbohydrates and sugars.

-During the diet, a process of oxidation of the fats that have remained in reserve in the body, over time, occurs as a result of a diet that has not been in accordance with the nutritional needs of the body.

-The body's natural mechanism is activated, in order to supply the lack of those foods that provide energy; carbohydrates and sugars, taking fats to convert them into energy for the body's functions.

-The consumption of large amounts of fats produces a feeling of fullness, increases energy and prevents the person from feeling the need to eat between meals, due to anxiety.

Difference between a traditional diet and the ketogenic diet

The main difference between traditional diets and the ketogenic diet is that the former uses carbohydrates and sugars as fuel, and in the ketogenic diet, the body makes use of fats to produce ketone bodies and consequently energy for the functioning of the body.

Combination of macronutrients

In the keto diet, the combination of macronutrients plays a fundamental role. Traditionally, in Western culture, a greater amount of carbohydrates has been included in meals, and a preference towards the consumption of sugars, with the keto diet, the metabolism is totally modified and the energy to live is taken from reserve fats.

A different diet produces a different response from the body.

Cooking techniques

The ketogenic diet, is flexible, does not force to use a specific technique of cooking, however, it is recommended to be careful during this process, to preserve the nutrients contained in food. In this sense, green vegetables should be steamed and care should be taken to preserve their fresh appearance. Many foods have their precise cooking point and others do not require this process.

Food selection and preparation

The recommended foods in the keto diet are preferably in their natural state. The quality of food is measured by its fresh appearance; this depends on the process of production, harvesting, transport and storage.

Although it is difficult to obtain all this information when choosing a food, it is important to pay attention to the color, texture and fresh appearance of the food.

You can keep them in compliance with the rules of hygiene and food preservation, for a maximum period of one week.

In the keto diet, it is important to measure the amounts of carbohydrates and avoid sugars, to obtain optimal results from the diet; the variation in the amounts directly influences the results.

Changes it produces in the metabolism

The human body responds to change in different ways, and in some people, it manifests itself differently than in others.

Among the positive changes generally observed during the keto diet are:

- Rapid weight loss.
- Release of increased sodium, through the kidneys.
- Change in the appearance of the stool.
- Production of more urine.
- Increased production of ketone bodies.
- Use of fat reserves as energy.
- Increased sweating.
- Use of fats instead of carbohydrates and sugars to produce the energy the body needs.

Chapter 2

How did Keto start? (Technology industry)

The ketogenic diet has its origin in fasting. Fasting has been recommended since ancient times to people suffering from any disease. The first results of the ketogenic diet demonstrated its effectiveness in neurological problems such as epilepsy and others.

In the archives of Hippocrates, the father of medicine, evidence has been found that fasting can contribute to the improvement of some pathology. The results of the ketogenic diet in ancient times are obtained empirically since there were no laboratories, and the results were obtained through observation.

Even in the bible, there are indications of the ketogenic diet, there are stories where fasting is recommended, to improve the health of the disciples. At this time the benefits of the ketogenic diet are empirically acquired and proven through observation.

At the beginning of the 21st century, scientists are discovering the potential of the ketogenic diet, on cases such as epilepsy, especially in children. In the world of fitness, the ketogenic diet is introduced as an excellent method of maintaining optimal physical condition, gaining great favor for its results.

After that moment, the ketogenic diet acquires great prestige and credibility, since the scientific community certifies its effectiveness and great benefits in general health.

The comparison of the effects of fasting and the ketogenic diet led scientists to conclude that the reduction of carbohydrates and a specific distribution of macronutrients results in the same health effects as fasting, with respect to ketone production. This discovery was wonderful, especially because it provides the necessary micronutrients and macronutrients and avoids exposing children in particular to great sacrifices.

It was widely used in the 1920s, 1930s and 1940s; however, with the evolution of technology and the growth of the pharmaceutical industry, the ketogenic diet was relegated to effective drugs to treat epilepsy, while at the same time appearing great detractors of the diet, in the scientific community.

It is important to note that at first because it was still under study, the keto diet was restrictive and imposed sacrifices for compliance, it was more practical for people, take a capsule and forget about the diet.

In the 2000- 2010 decade, the keto diet was held only in the fitness world, as a method of weight loss. There have been diets related to the keto diet; however, groups of orthodox scientists are responsible for rating these diets negatively.

An emblematic case occurred to the boy Charlie, his experience with the keto diet in relation to his illness was very positive, it showed considerable improvement, it was known worldwide and this case gave a great impulse again to the ketogenic diet.

Today it is one of the favorite diets for weight loss; conditions of many typical diseases of modernity such as diabetes type II, there are ongoing studies on the effect and progress in complex diseases such as cancer, cardiovascular and neurodegenerative diseases.

The ketogenic diet is an effective and safe strategy to show off a stylish physical appearance and regain health.

Why are dieticians against it?

Some professionals who oppose the ketogenic diet base their theory on the ketogenic diet, considering that a high-fat diet has an incidence of cardiovascular problems. However, the ketogenic diet is clear by pointing out the foods that are allowed and those that should be restricted, in its recommendations and puts the recommendation of healthy fats, especially unsaturated and monounsaturated fats, contained in food in the foreground.

There will always be detractors of the keto diet, especially because of the success of this diet on the metabolism and the improvement in the quality of life of people, which it has been shown to have. This phenomenon is due to market interests, competition, supply and demand, which is part of the fierce mercantilism, which seeks the enrichment of few compared to the welfare of the majority.

Chapter 3

Side effects

Generally, the ketogenic diet does not produce major side effects, which in any way jeopardize compliance with the diet and the person's health. In some cases, the person experiences small signs that their body has entered a state of ketosis and it manifests itself through small colds, dizziness, nausea, thirst, among other symptoms.

Most people, who adopt the keto diet, claim to have no side effects.

After starting the keto diet, you may start to feel some symptoms, which are positive, since they indicate that your diet is having an effect on your body.

How do you know if your body has entered a state of ketosis?

The body indicates when it has been inducted into a ketosis state by the keto diet.

It is important to be aware of changes in your body, such as:

* Keto flu

Keto flu occurs during the body's period of adaptation to dietary changes, just as it begins to burn off stored fat due to the ketosis-induced state the body is in through the ketogenic diet. Keto flu can be confused with a common cold, as its symptoms are similar.

* Taste in the mouth and a smell characteristic of the fruit

* Intense thirst and dry skin

* Presence of ketones in urine and blood (observable through laboratory tests)

* Weight loss

* Low energy, due to low sugar and carbohydrate intake

* Fatigue

* Decay or lack of interest in doing everyday tasks

* Metabolic acidosis which can cause diarrhea, vomiting, nausea and others.

The symptoms described above are mild, remain while the period of adaptation of the metabolism to the ketogenic diet occurs, and disappear briefly without the need for medication.

**In some cases, it is advisable to apply some tricks that correct in a healthy and immediate way, these symptoms, for example:

Ketosis excess high levels of ketone in the blood are balanced by consuming small amounts of carbohydrates.

Keto flu will disappear on its own while the body's adaptation to the diet occurs, however, it is advisable to stay hydrated, take sodium, magnesium and potassium supplements, as well as eating enough foods containing Omega-3s.

To reduce the symptoms of keto flu, it is recommended to drink some water with a little salt, if necessary 3 times a day, until the symptoms improve.

How to measure ketones in the blood?

If you want to measure the ketones in your body, you can do it through different techniques:

- Blood test

- Urine test

- Reagent strips you can get on the market.

Chapter 4

Benefits

Among the most important benefits of the keto diet is:

- Increased energy

- Mental clarity

- Weight loss

- Improved health

- Disease prevention

- Strengthens the immune system

- Reduces the risk of cardiovascular disease.

- Higher performance

- Balances insulin levels

- Increases positive emotions and good mood.

- Strength and physical performance.

It is important to note that to obtain the benefits of the ketogenic diet for the body, carbohydrate consumption should be reduced to less than 50 grams per day. That is the equivalent of a slice of bread and avoids the consumption of sugars, some fruits with high fructose content, tubers and legumes

Chapter 5

35 Nutritious and delicious recipes from Keto, easy to prepare with 5 ingredients and in only 15 minutes.

Soups

1. Corn and Tomato Soup

Kcal (100g) 282.98/ **Protein (100)** 18.5/ **Carbohydrates(100g)** 35.14/ **Fats (100g)** 27.06

Ingredients
- 2 Tomatoes finely cubed
- 4 Crushed garlic
- 1 Red onion finely chopped
- 1 Can of sweet corn, drained
- Coconut oil

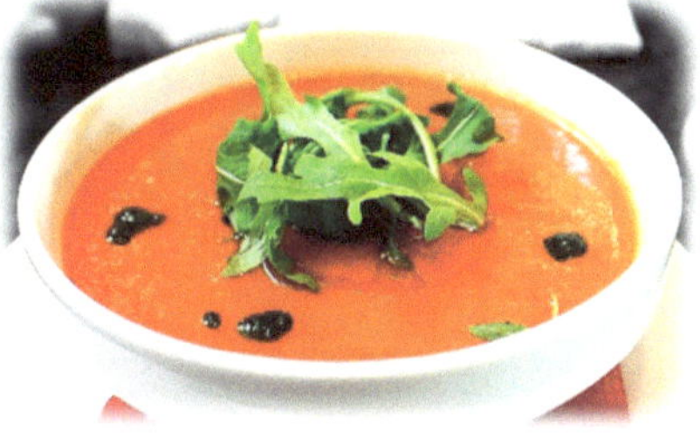

Preparation
In a hot frying pan over medium-high heat, place oil with tomato, onion, garlic and sauté until golden brown. Add sweet corn, sauté with the season to taste for a few minutes, take to the blender glass and process it with water until a creamy texture is obtained. Serve and decorate to taste.

2. Sweet Corn Cream

Kcal (100g) 114.9/ **Protein (100)** 13.7/ **Carbohydrates(100g)** 27.14/ **Fats (100g)** 26.25

Ingredients

- 1 Can of sweet corn, drained
- 1 Onion finely chopped
- 3 Crushed garlic
- 1 Yellow sweet pepper chopped
- Olive oil

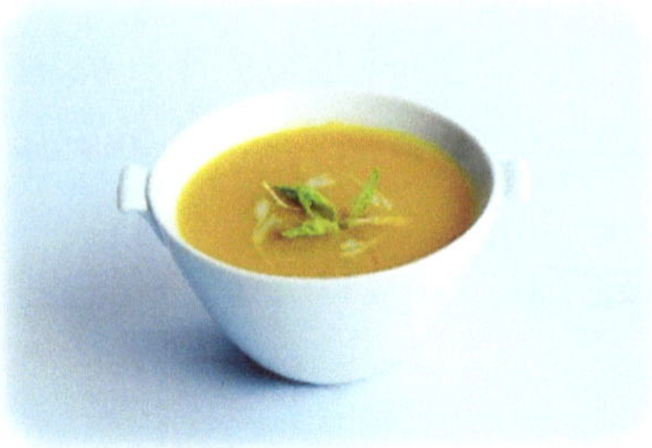

Preparation

In a hot over medium-high heat, place oil, onion, sweet pepper, garlic and sauté until golden brown. Add sweet corn; mix with the season to taste and place all in a blender glass. Process it with a few oil and water until a creamy texture is obtained. Serve and decorate to taste.

3. Beetroot Cream

Kcal (100g) 104.58/ **Protein (100)** 7.1/ **Carbohydrates(100g)** 17.4/ **Fats (100g)** 40.0

Ingredients

- 3 Beetroot cubed
- 1 Carrot shredded
- 2 Bay leaf
- 1 Tbsp of shredded ginger
- Coconut oil

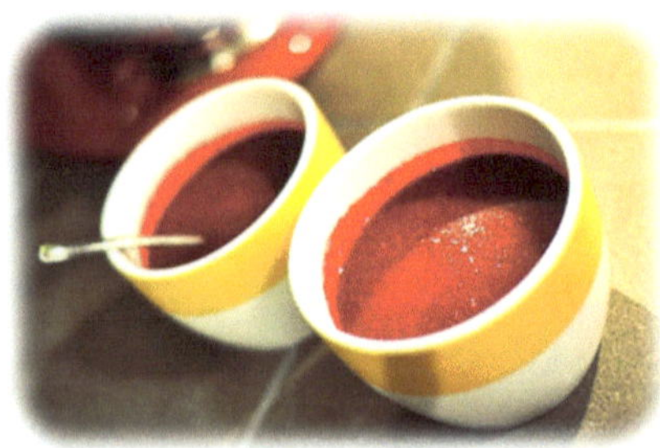

Preparation

In a pot over high heat, place oil, beetroot, carrot, ginger and sauté it until golden brown. Add hot water until cover the half, bay leaf with the season to taste, cover with a lid and cook a few minutes. Process it with an immersion blender, serve and decorate to taste.

4. Light Artichoke Broth

Kcal (100g) 52.12/ **Protein (100)** 7.1/ **Carbohydrates(100g)** 13/ **Fats (100g)** 40.0

Ingredients

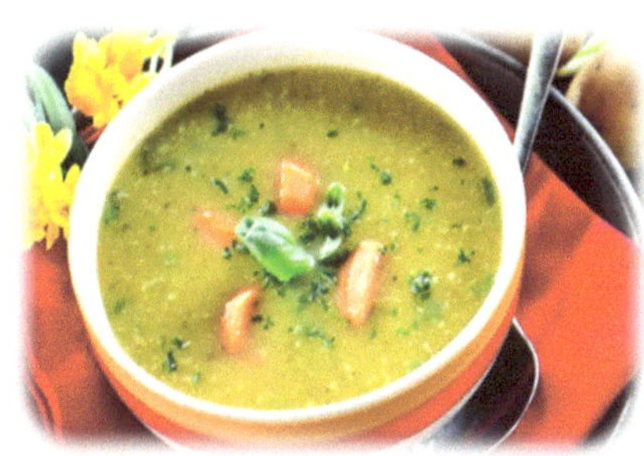

- 400g of cleaned artichokes
- 2 Red onion finely chopped
- 3 Crushed garlic
- 2 Tbsp of paprika
- Olive oil

Preparation

Remove the leaves of the artichoke and set aside. In a hot wok over medium-high heat, place oil with onion, artichoke, garlic, and paprika, season to taste and sauté for 5 minutes. Add 2 cups of hot water, cover with a lid, and cook for 10 minutes. Remove from heat, serve and decorate to taste.

5. Light Detox Broth

Kcal (100g) 118.7/ **Protein (100)** 2.25/ **Carbohydrates(100g)** 20.0/ **Fats (100g)** 26.12

Ingredients

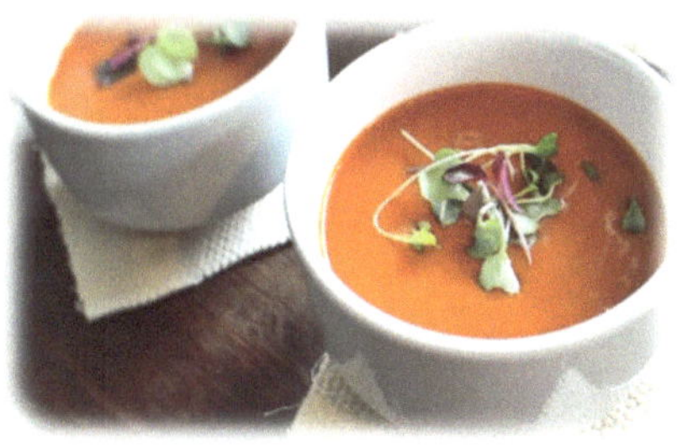

- 1 Leek finely chopped
- 1 Celery stalk finely chopped
- 1 Shredded carrot
- 2 Red onion finely chopped
- Sesame oil

Preparation

In a hot frying pan over medium-high heat, place oil with onion, leek and sauté until golden brown. Add celery, carrot and sauté until golden brown. Take to the blender glass with 2 cups of hot water, process it until homogenize, place in heat until boil and let rest a few minutes. Serve and decorate to taste.

6. Fat-Remover Soup

Kcal (100g) 56.25/ **Protein (100)** 3.5/ **Carbohydrates(100g)** 25.0/ **Fats (100g)** 1.0

Ingredients

- 2 Red onion chopped
- 1 Celery stalk chopped
- 1 Sweet pepper chopped
- 1 Cup of spinach
- 2 Bay leaf

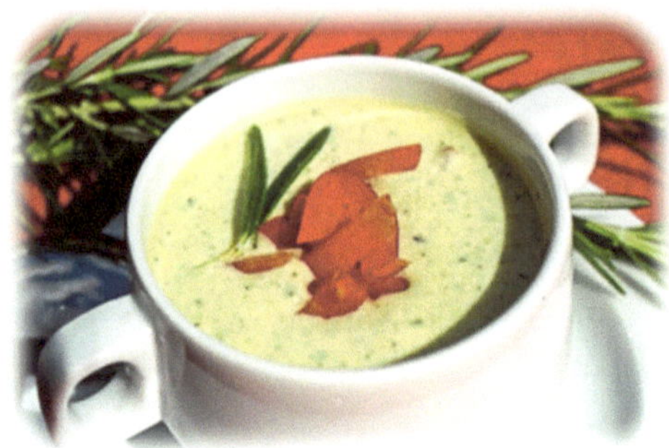

Preparation

In a pot with 400ml of boiling water over high heat, place all ingredients and cook for 10 minutes. Season to taste, serve and decorate to taste. Or place all in the blender glass and process it until homogenize, serve and decorate to taste.

7. Roast Vegetable Cream

Kcal (100g) 225/ **Protein (1003.5g)**/ **Carbohydrates(100g)** 25.0/ **Fats (100g)** 20.7

Ingredients

- 1 Carrot Shredded
- 400g of pumpkin diced
- 1 Leek finely chopped
- 1 Zucchini cubed
- Olive oil

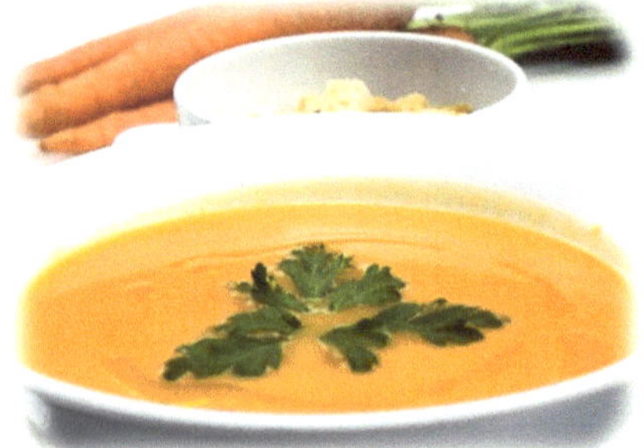

Preparation

In a heat-resistant tray place all ingredients, bathe with olive oil and season with prefer aromatic herbs. Take to the preheated oven at 400°F /200°C for 8 – 12 minutes. Place all in the blender glass and process it with water until a light texture is obtained. Serve, decorate to taste and consume hot.

8. Fresh Energetic Soup

Kcal (100g) 221.0/ **Protein (100g)** 2.25/ **Carbohydrates(100g)** 13.0/ **Fats (100g)** 20.7

Ingredients

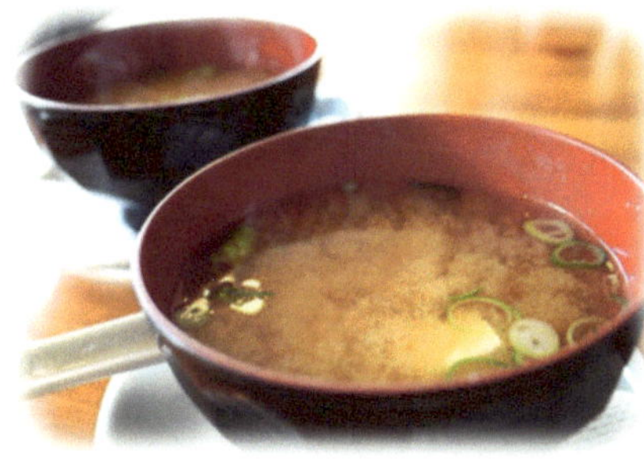

- 2 Celery stalks finely chopped
- 1 Red onion finely chopped
- 4 Crushed garlic
- 1 Tbsp of paprika
- Coconut oil

Preparation

In a pot over medium-high heat, place all ingredients and sauté until golden brown. Add 2 cups of hot water, season to taste, cover with a lid and cook for 5 – 10 minutes. Serve passing it for a strainer and decorate to taste. Also, you can process it with a blender, serve and decorate to taste.

9. Chicken Breast Consommé

Kcal (100g) 229.6/ **Protein (100g)** 7.5/ **Carbohydrates(100g)** 10.6/ **Fats (100g)** 33.12

Ingredients

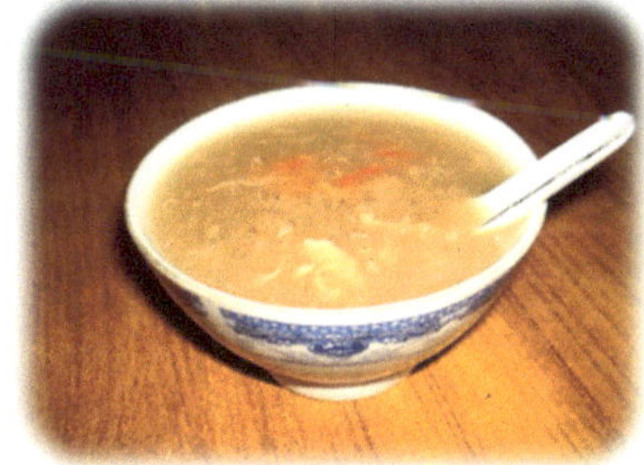

- 1 Chicken breast diced
- 1 Red onion finely chopped
- 5 Crushed garlic
- ½ Carrot shredded

Preparation

In a pot over medium-high heat, place oil with chicken and sauté until golden brown; then remove from heat and reserve. In the same pot, place oil, onion, garlic, carrot and sauté until golden brown. Add chicken, 2 cups of boiling water, season to taste, cover with a lid and cook for 7 – 10 minutes. Remove from heat, serve and decorate to taste.

9. Leek and Chicken Cream

Kcal (100g)247.98/ **Protein (100g)**7.89/ **Carbohydrates(100g)**11.94/ **Fats (100g)** 33.02

Ingredients

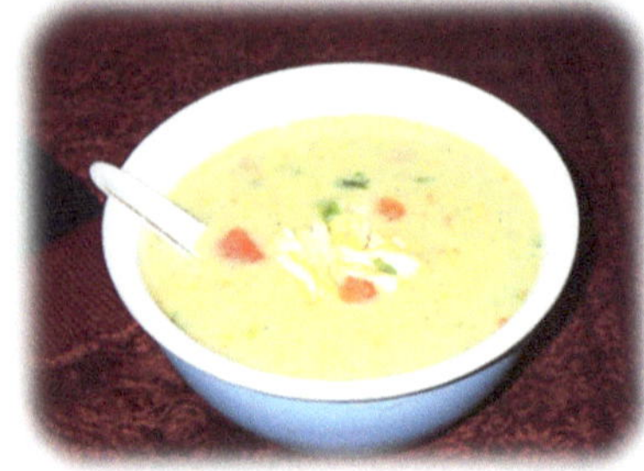

- 2 Leeks finely chopped
- 1 Chicken breast diced
- 1 Carrot shredded
- A cup of hot chicken broth
- Coconut oil

Preparation

In a pot over medium-high heat, place oil with chicken and sauté until golden brown. Remove from heat and reserve. In the same pot, place oil with leek, carrot and sauté until golden brown. Add chicken, season to taste, add broth, cover with the lid and cook for 10 minutes. Place in the blender glass, process until a creamy texture is obtained, serve and decorate to taste.

Mains

1. Chicken Breast in Oriental Sauce

Kcal (100g) 232.1/ **Protein (100g)** 11.12/ **Carbohydrates(100g)** 1.0/ **Fats (100g)** 59.75

Ingredients

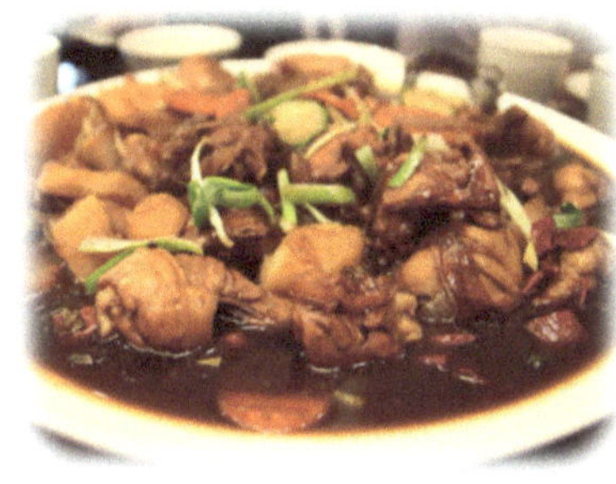

- 1 Chicken breast diced
- ½ Cup of oriental sauce
- 30g of butter
- ½ Cup of white wine
- Olive oil

Preparation

In a hot frying pan over medium-high heat, place butter with oil, chicken and sauté until golden brown. Add oriental sauce, wine cover with the lid and cook for 5 – 7 minutes. Add season to taste, mix and set aside. Serve in a bowl, decorate to taste and accompany with brown rice.

2. Mushroom with Pork Sautéed Au Gratin

Kcal (100g) 270.8/ **Protein (100g)** 10.5/ **Carbohydrates(100g)** 2.92/ **Fats (100g)** 30.72

Ingredients

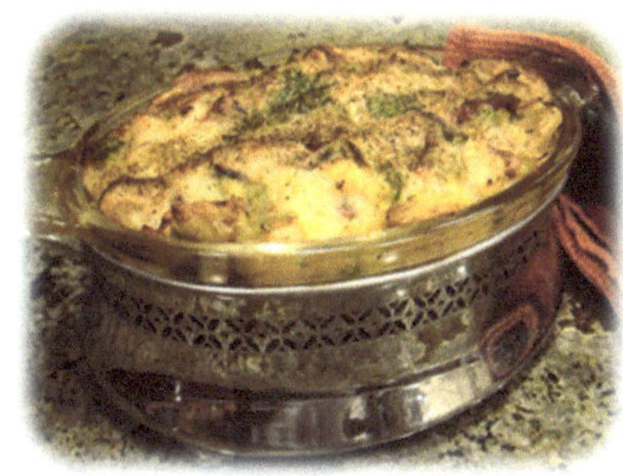

- 1 Can of mushroom, drained
- 100g of mozzarella shredded
- 20ml of red wine
- 120g of ground pork
- Coconut oil

Preparation

In a hot wok over medium-high heat, place oil with pork and sauté until golden brown. Add mushroom with wine, season to taste and sauté for 5 minutes. Reduce to medium-low heat, place in the top the mozzarella, cover with the lid and cook until cheese is melted. Remove from heat, let rest a few minutes, serve and decorate.

3. Lettuce Mix with Pork

Kcal (100g) 232.1/ **Protein (100g)** 6.62/ **Carbohydrates(100g)** 5.4/ **Fats (100g)** 26.1

Ingredients

- 400g of ground pork
- 1 Pack of 5-lettuce mix
- 2 Tbsp of paprika
- 4 Crushed garlic
- Canola oil

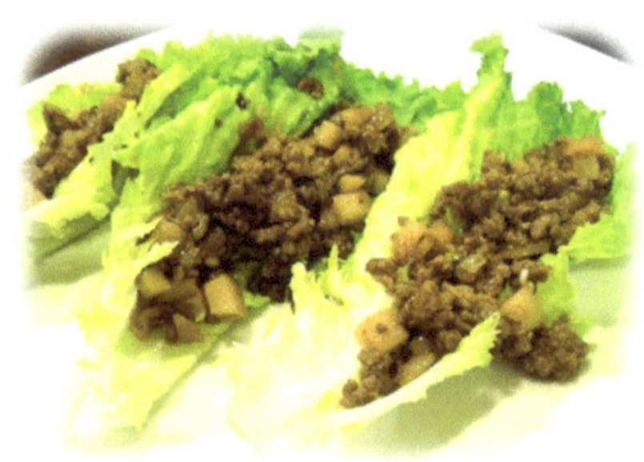

Preparation

In a hot frying pan over medium-high heat, place oil, garlic, paprika and sauté quickly. Add pork, season to taste and sauté until golden brown, mixing and separating all meat until is lump-free. Remove from heat, and place it with the 5-lettuce mix, mix all, serve and decorate to taste.

4. Pork with Julienne Mix & Mustard

Kcal (100g) 274.4/ **Protein (100g)** 9.65/ **Carbohydrates(100g)** 2.0/ **Fats (100g)** 34.67

Ingredients

- 300g of pork loin diced
- 5 Crushed garlic
- 1 Pack of julienne mix
- 3 Tbsp of mustard
- Olive oil

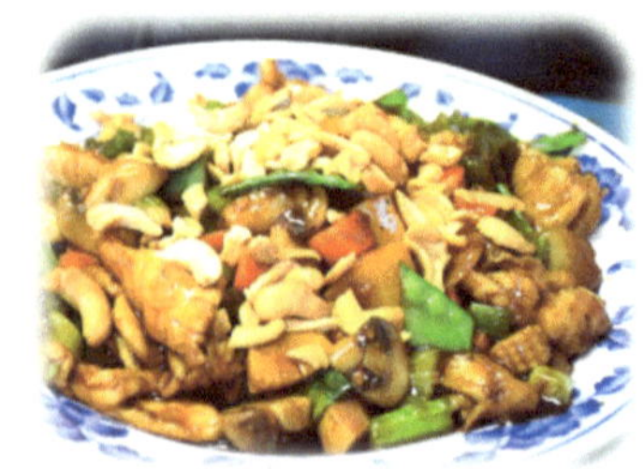

Preparation

In a hot frying pan, over medium-high heat, place oil with pork and seal for all sides. Remove from heat and reserve. In the same frying pan, place oil with garlic, julienne mix and sauté until golden brown. Add pork, mustard, season to taste, ½ cup of hot water and cook until the liquid reduces. Serve and decorate.

5. Dressed Salmon in Papillote

Kcal (100g) 70.8/ **Protein (100g)** 6.86/ **Carbohydrates(100g)** 0.56/ **Fats (100g)** 4.0

Ingredients

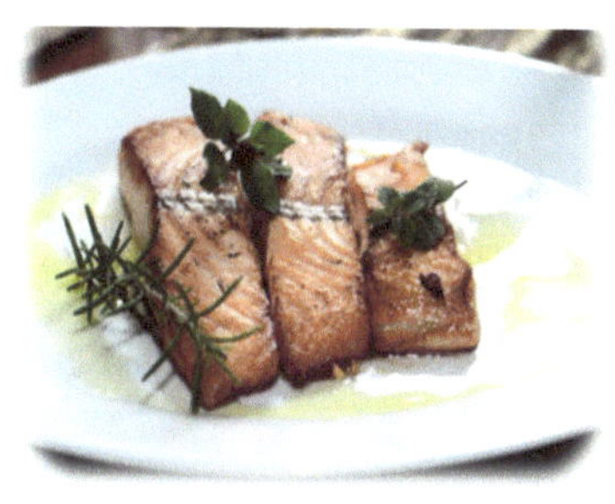

- 250g of salmon
- 5 Crushed garlic
- 10ml of pink wine
- 1 Red onion in julienne
- Juice of 1 lemon

Preparation

Grab 1 sheet of paraffin paper, place the salmon in center and fold the 4 extremes forming an envelope. Add to salmon the garlic, onion, wine, lemon juice, and closet the envelope, without leave any opening. Place it in a heat-resistant tray, and take it to the preheated oven at 380°F/185°C for 12 – 15 minutes. Remove from oven, open carefully the envelope, serve and decorate.

6. Aromatized Chicken with Salad

Kcal (100g) 218.2/ **Protein (100g)** 6.33/ **Carbohydrates(100g)** 3.03/ **Fats (100g)** 30.55

Ingredients

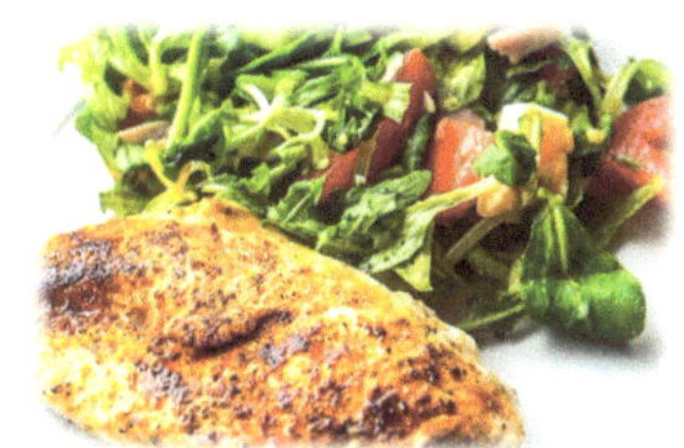

- 1 Chicken breast
- 2 Tbsp of butter
- 2 Sticks of thyme
- 1 Tbsp of paprika
- 1 Vegetable salad kit

Preparation

In a bowl place butter, leaves of thyme, paprika and mix until homogenize. Season the chicken to taste, cover it with the flavored butter, and place it a hot frying pan over medium-high heat. Cover with the lid; cook for 5 – 8 minutes each side. Serve with vegetable salad; bathe with butter in the frying pan and decorate to taste.

7. Beef Salad Roll

Kcal (100g) 83.1/ **Protein (100g)** 21.1/ **Carbohydrates(100g)** 2.0/ **Fats (100g)** 7.2

Ingredients

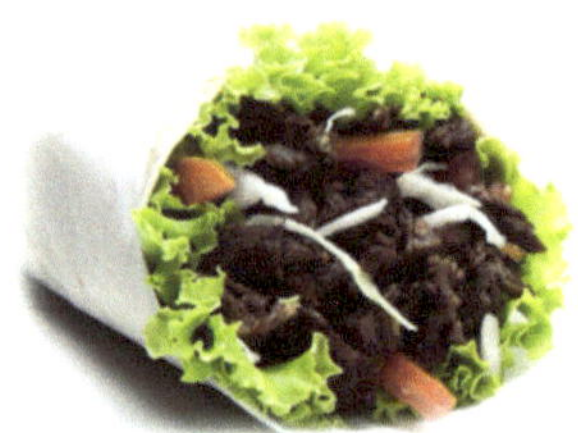

- 300g of beef in strips
- 50ml of oriental sauce
- Prefer low-carb dressing
- Olive oil
- 1 Pack of American salad mix

Preparation

In a bowl place American salad, olive oil, mix and reserve. In a hot frying pan over medium-high heat, place olive oil with beef and sauté until golden brown. Add oriental sauce, season to taste, mix and cook for 5 – 8 minutes. In a sheet of paraffin paper, place salad, dressing, and sautéed beef, and roll it. Serve accompanied with dressing.

8. Pork Sirloin with Coriander Sauce

Kcal (100g) 226.2/ **Protein (100g)** 9.66/ **Carbohydrates(100g)** 4.33/ **Fats (100g)** 32.87

Ingredients

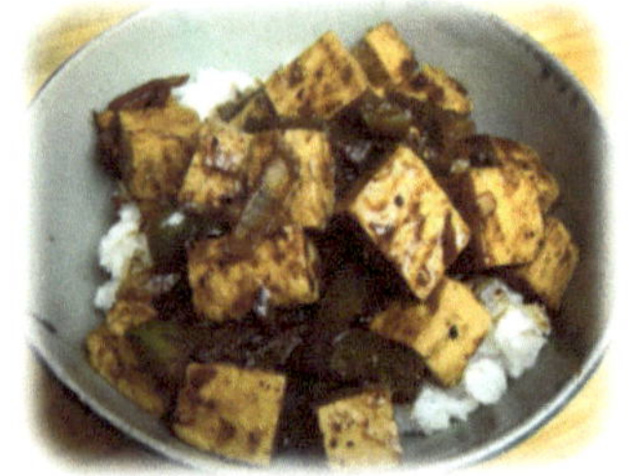

- 300g of pork sirloin diced
- A cup of coriander leaves
- Provencal herbs
- 15ml of oriental sauce
- Olive oil

Preparation

In the blender glass, place oriental sauce, a little of olive oil, coriander leaves, and a little water, then process all until homogenized. In a hot frying pan over medium-high heat, place oil with sirloin and sauté until golden brown. Add the previously processed coriander, Provencal herbs, season to taste, cover with the lid and cook for 10 minutes. Serve and decorate to taste.

9. Aromatic Hake with Salad Mix

Kcal (100g) 252.2/ **Protein (100g)** 5.83/ **Carbohydrates(100g)** 2.72/ **Fats (100g)** 28.93

Ingredients

- 1 Hake filet
- Juice of 2 lemons
- 2 Tbsp of aromatic herbs
- 1 Pack of salad kit
- Olive oil

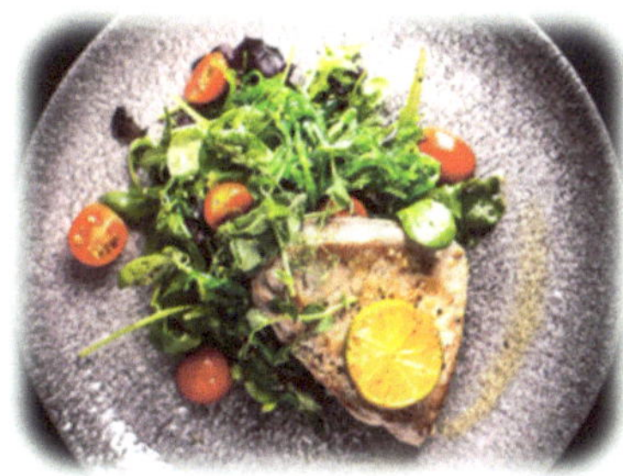

Preparation

Grab a sheet of paraffin paper, place in center the hake and fold the 4 extremes forming an envelope for the oven. Add lemon juice, a little of olive oil and aromatic herbs to hake. Close the envelope without leaving any opening and take to the preheated oven at 390ºF/195ºC for 6 – 10 minutes. Open the envelope with caution to not to burn yourself with hot vapors, serve with the 5-lettuce mix.

10. Cauliflower Veggie Pizza

Kcal (100g) 278.2/ **Protein (100g)** 8.74/ **Carbohydrates(100g)** 2.52/ **Fats (100g)** 33.9

Ingredients

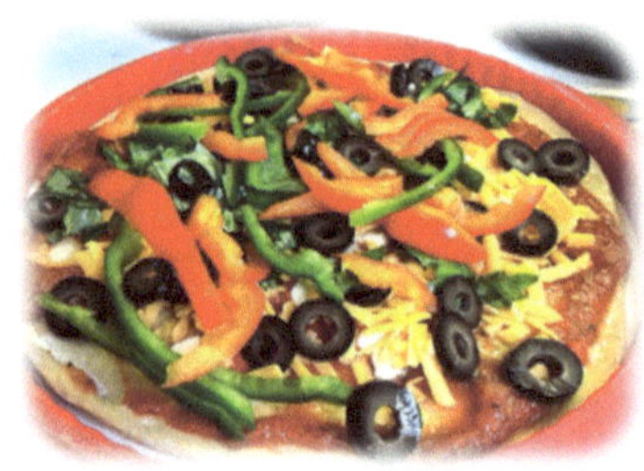

- 1 Cauliflower shelled
- 3 Eggs
- 150g of cheddar shredded
- Vegetal filling to taste
- Olive oil

Preparation

In a pot with salted boiling water, place cauliflower and cook for 1 – 2 minutes. Drain it and place in a food processor. Add eggs, cheddar, and process it until firm dough is formed. Stretch it in a heat-resistant tray to taste and take to the preheated oven at 390ºF/195ºC for 5 – 8 minutes. Fill to taste, varnish the boards with olive oil and cook 5 minutes. Let rest a few moments, decorate to taste, cut and serve.

Desserts

1. Sweet Potato & Dry Fruits Bread

Kcal (100g) 228.6/ **Protein (100g)** 7.6/ **Carbohydrates(100g)** 24.42/ **Fats (100g)** 12.26

Ingredients

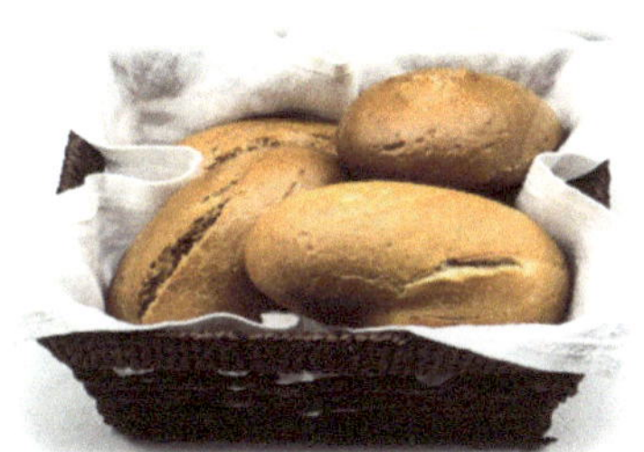

- 500g of cooked sweet potato
- ½ Tsp of stevia powder
- 2 Cups of chickpea flour
- 1 Tbsp of baking soda
- A cup of dry fruits chopped

Preparation

Place the sweet potato in a bowl and crush it forming a puree.
Place in the bowl the rest of ingredients and 1 and ½ cup of water,
and process it with an electric kneader until firm dough is obtained.
Stir and cut to taste. Form spheres from the dough, and place those
in a heat-resistant tray previously prepared with paraffin paper.
Take to the preheated oven at 380°F/185°C for 10 – 12 minutes, let
rest and serve.

2. Sweet Pineapple in Ron

Kcal (100g) 142.6/ **Protein (100g)** 0.2/**Carbohydrates(100g)** 27.6/ **Fats (100g)** 0.1

Ingredients

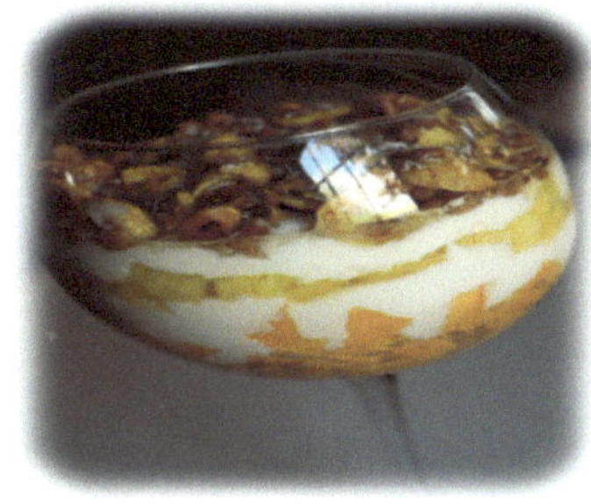

- 1 Pineapple cubed
- A cup of white Ron
- ½ Tsp of stevia powder
- 2 Cups of orange juice
- 1 Vanilla pod

Preparation

Cut the vanilla pod in halves, scrape the seeds and reserve. In a pot over medium-high heat, place Ron, stevia, orange juice, vanilla pod and seeds, and cook without leaving mixing until golden brown. Add pineapple and cook for 10 – 15 minutes mixing periodically. Serve fresh or cold with yogurt, ice cream or to taste.

3. Cheese and Cream Keto Cake

Kcal (100g)193.2/ **Protein (100g)** 18.08/**Carbohydrates(100g)** 18.34/**Fats (100g)** 11.59

Ingredients

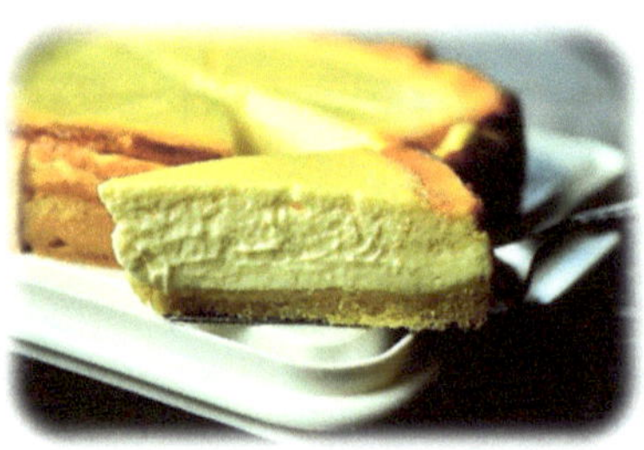

- 350g of keto cookies
- 300g of cream cheese
- 5 Eggs
- 150g of milk cream
- ½ Tsp of stevia powder

Preparation

Grab the cookies and crush them to get sand from cookies. In a bowl, place eggs, cheese, stevia and mix until homogenize. In another bowl place milk cream and beat with an electric whisk until mounted cream is obtained. Add to eggs and mix in enveloping form until homogenize. Cover the bottom of a prepared cake mold with cookies, add the mixture of eggs and milk cream, and take to the preheated oven at 400ºF/200ºC for 8 – 12 minutes. Remove from heat, let rest, cut and serve to taste.

4. Delight of Cauliflower Rice and Coconut

Kcal (100g) 319.0/ **Protein (100g)** 3.45/ **Carbohydrates(100g)** 17.84/ **Fats (100g)** 26.64

Ingredients

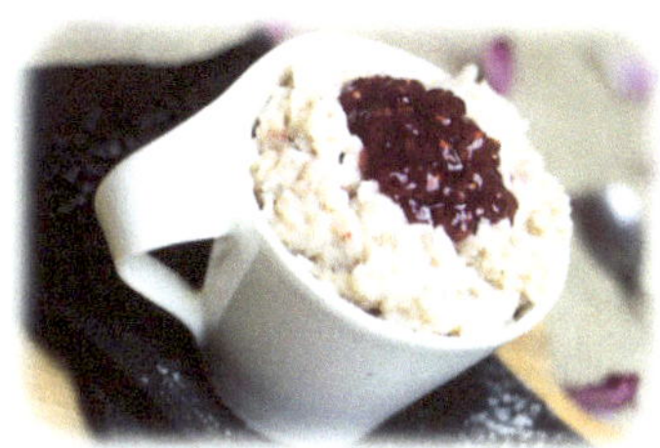

- 1 Cauliflower shelled
- A cup of coconut milk
- A cup of toasted shredded coconut
- 1 Can of gluten-free condensed milk
- 2 Tbsp of cinnamon

Preparation

Place the cauliflower in the food processor and process it for 3 – 5 minutes to obtain very small grains. In a pot over medium-high heat, place coconut milk, cinnamon, coconut, condensed milk and cook mixing until a creamy texture is obtained. Add cauliflower and mix for a few minutes. Let rest, serve fresh or cold from the fridge and decorate to taste.

5. Sweet Keto Donuts

Kcal (100g) 356.98/ **Protein(100g)** 6.01/ **Carbohydrates(100g)** 26.64/ **Fats (100g)** 42.1

Ingredients

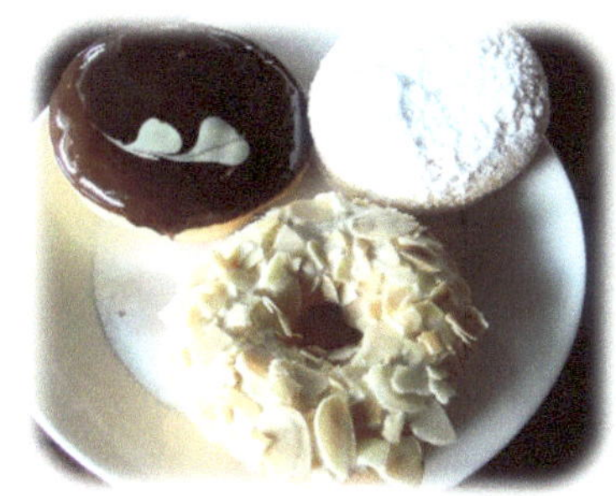

- A cup of chickpea flour
- ½ Tsp of stevia powder
- A cup of soymilk
- 40g of butter
- Olive oil

Preparation

In a bowl, place all ingredients and mix with an electric kneader until firm dough is formed. Grab portions to taste, make thin discs, make a hole in the center and place those in a frying pan with hot oil at medium-high heat. Let golden brown the discs for all sides, cover with dark chocolate, mounted cream or to taste, let cold and serve.

6. Chocolate Fritters

Kcal (100g) 450.4/ **Protein(100g)** 6.07/**Carbohydrates(100g)** 35.3/**Fats (100g)** 32.9

Ingredients

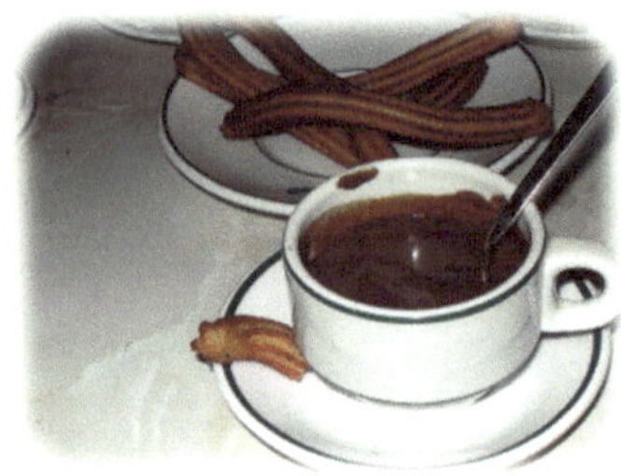

- 40g of cocoa powder
- A cup of chickpea flour
- ½ Tsp of stevia powder
- A cup of coconut milk
- 50g of melted butter

Preparation

In a bowl place chickpea flour and cocoa powder passing by a strainer. Add the rest of ingredients and mix with an electric whisk until firm dough is formed. Grab portions to form cylinders of 10 – 15cm and 2cm of thickness. Place it in a previously prepared heat-resistant tray and take it to the preheated oven at 400°F/200°C for 5 – 12 minutes. Bathe with dark chocolate or to taste and serve.

7. Dark Chocolate Stove Bread

Kcal (100g) 305.8/ **Protein(100g)** 10.49/**Carbohydrates(100g)** 25.34/**Fats (100g)** 21.44

Ingredients

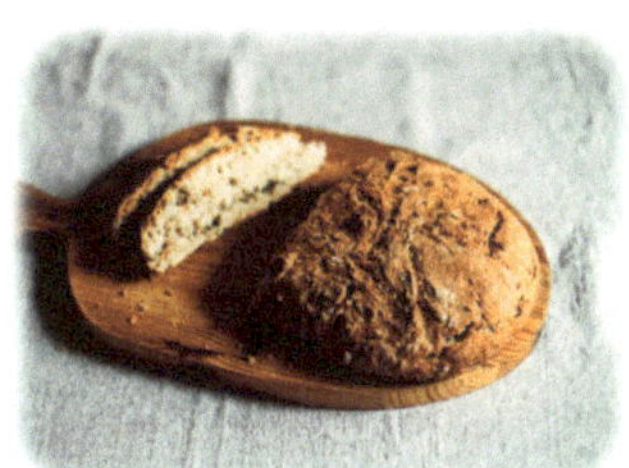

- 100g of melted dark chocolate
- 300g of chickpea flour
- 3 Eggs
- 1 Tbsp of baking soda
- ½ Tsp of stevia powder

Preparation

In a bowl place all ingredients with 2 cups of warm water and mix with hands until firm dough is formed. Take portions of 50 – 70g of dough, form discs and place those in a hot non-stick frying pan over low heat. Press lightly down the discs, cover with the lid and cook 3 minutes for each side twice. Remove from heat and serve with milk or to taste.

8. Avocado Keto Brownie

Kcal (100g) 299/ **Protein(100g)** 7.9/**Carbohydrates(100g)** 23.26/**Fats (100g)** 20.75

Ingredients

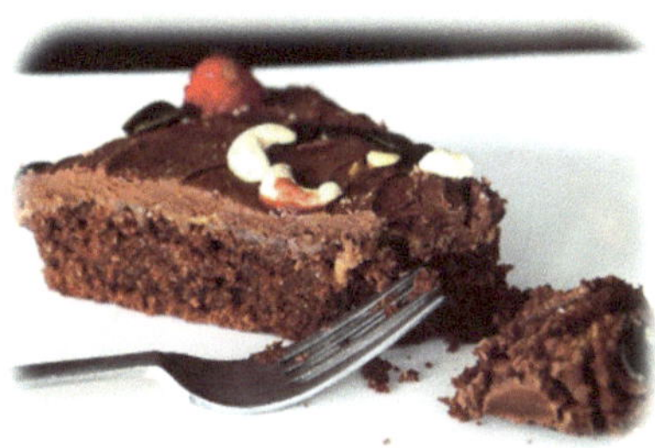

- 150g of melted dark chocolate
- 1 Avocado
- 4 Eggs
- ½ Tsp of stevia powder
- 50g of cocoa powder]

Preparation

Cut the avocado in halves, remove the seed, and place in a bowl the pulp. Add the rest of ingredients to avocado and mix with an electric whisk until homogenize. Pour the mixture in a previously prepared heat-resistant tray and take it to the preheated oven at 400°F/200°C for 10 – 15 minutes. Let rest, cut in squares, and serve with vanilla ice cream or to taste.

9. Almond Fluffy Cupcake

Kcal (100g) 272.4/ **Protein(100g)** 14.01/**Carbohydrates(100g)** 20.25/**Fats (100g)** 36.7

Ingredients

- 4 Eggs
- A cup of almond flour
- 1 Tbsp of baking soda
- 1 Tbsp of xanthan gum
- ½ Tsp of stevia powder

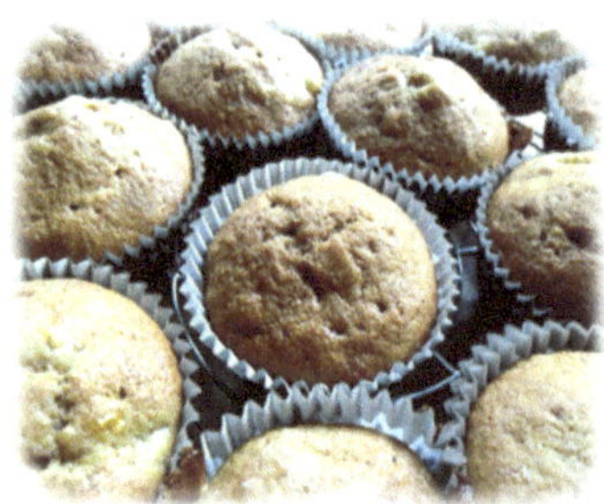

Preparation

Place the almond flour, baking soda and xanthan gum in a strainer, and mix passing through it. In a bowl place eggs, stevia, and beat with an electric whisk until gets creamy. Add the flour mix in parts, mixing in enveloping form until homogenize. Pour it in a previously prepared cupcake mold and take it to the preheated oven at 400°F/200°C for 5 – 10 minutes. Remove from heat, let rest a few minutes, and serve to taste.

10. Cappuccino Flavour Cupcake

Kcal (100g) 342.4/ **Protein(100g)** 14.92/**Carbohydrates(100g)** 24.96/**Fats (100g)** 11.47

Ingredients

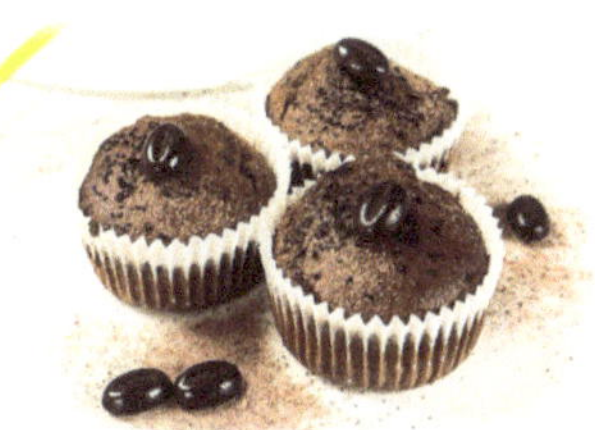

- 50ml of black coffee
- A cup of gluten-free condensed milk
- 4 Eggs
- 30ml of brandy
- 300g of chickpea flour

Preparation

In a bowl place condensed milk, brandy, flour, coffee and mix until homogenize and set aside. In another bowl place eggs and beat with an electric whisk until gets creamy. Add the beaten eggs to the previous mixture of flour and mix in enveloping form until homogenize. Add mixture to previously prepared cupcake mold, decorate to taste and take it to the preheated oven at 400°F/200°C for 6 – 12 minutes. Let rest a few moments and serve to taste.

Snack

1. Cauliflower Croquettes

Kcal (100g) 337.2/ **Protein(100g)** 10.66/**Carbohydrates(100g)** 12.68/**Fats (100g)** 26.28

Ingredients

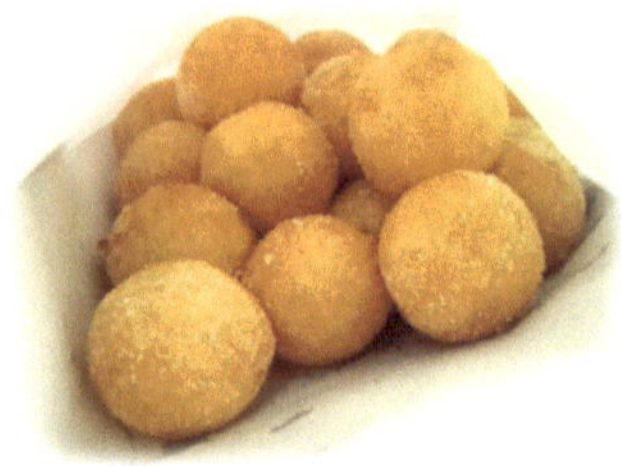

- 1 Cauliflower shelled
- 4 Eggs
- 40g of paprika
- A cup of chickpea flour
- Olive oil

Preparation

In a pot with salted boiling water, place cauliflower and cook for 2 – 4 minutes. Drain the cauliflower and place it in a food processor with eggs, paprika, chickpea flour, season to taste and process it until dough is obtained. Form small ovals from the dough and place it in the frying pan with hot oil. Cook until golden brown for all sides, remove from heat and serve with prefer dip.

2. Crispy Mozzarella Sticks

Kcal (100g) 255.1/ **Protein(100g)** 12.44/**Carbohydrates(100g)** 16.20/**Fats (100g)** 36.08

Ingredients

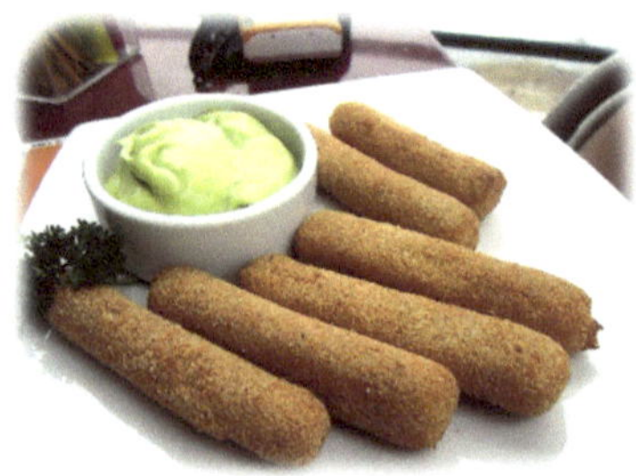

- 300g of mozzarella in sticks
- ½ Cup of chickpea flour
- 300g of almond flour
- 30g of paprika
- Olive oil

Preparation

In a bowl place chickpea flour, paprika and mix with warm water until a creamy texture is obtained; then place the almond flour in a dish. Grab the mozzarella sticks, bathe in the chickpea flour mix, then pass for almond flour, place the stick in a frying pan with hot oil and cook until golden brown. Remove from heat and serve alone or with prefer dip.

3. Battered Vegetables

Kcal (100g) 368.0/ **Protein(100g)** 8.1/**Carbohydrates(100g)** 24.56/**Fats (100g)** 25.64

Ingredients

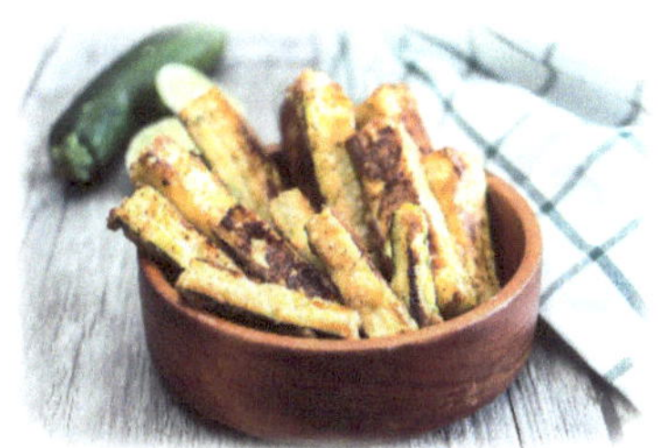

- Vegetables to taste in sticks
- A cup of chickpea flour
- 2 Tbsp of paprika
- 2 Tbsp of garlic powder
- Olive oil

Preparation

In a bowl, place chickpea flour, paprika, garlic powder, and mix vigorously with cold water until gets creamy. Bathe the vegetable sticks in the mixture, and then take those to the frying pan with hot oil and cook a few moments, until golden brown.

4. Buffalo-Style Cauliflower Trees

Kcal (100g) 154.6/ **Protein(100g)** 5.27/**Carbohydrates(100g)** 29.75/**Fats (100g)** 3.83

Ingredients

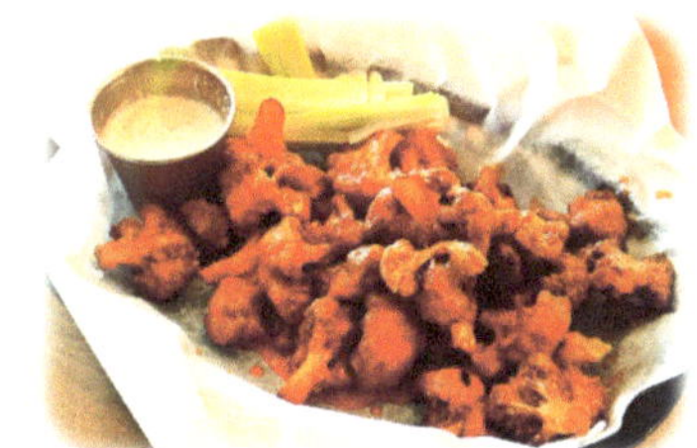

- 1 Cauliflower shelled
- A cup of chickpea flour
- ½ Tsp of stevia powder
- 1 Cup of beer
- Tabasco sauce to taste

Preparation

In a pot with salted boiling water, place cauliflower and cook for 2 – 4 minutes; then drain it and reserve. In a bowl place, the rest of the ingredients and beat vigorously until homogenize. Add to the mixture the cauliflower and mix to impregnate all cauliflower. Place the cauliflower in a previously prepared heat-resistant tray and take it to the preheated oven at 390°F/195°C for 3 – 5 minutes. Remove from heat, let rest a few minutes and serve to taste.

5. Battered Mango

Kcal (100g) 126.22/ **Protein(100g)** 7.67/**Carbohydrates(100g)** 17.58/**Fats (100g)** 6.91

Ingredients

- 2 Mangos
- A cup of chickpea flour
- ½ Tsp of stevia powder
- A cup of carbonated water
- Olive oil

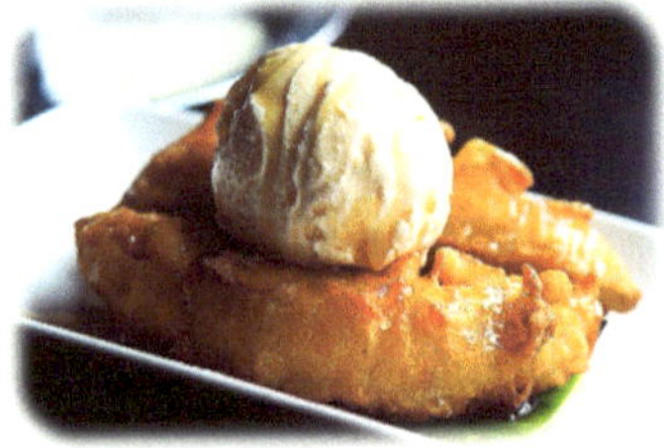

Preparation

In a bowl, place flour, carbonated water, stevia and mix until gets creamy. Peel and cut the mangos in wedges, bathe it in the mixture and place those in a frying pan with hot oil. Cook until golden brown for all sides, remove from heat and put those over napkins. Serve with a ball of ice cream, melted dark chocolate, mounted cream, or fruit syrup, or to taste.

Chapter 6

Food for consumption in the keto?

- Avocado

- Coconut

- Eggs

- Nuts

- Green leafy vegetables

- Orange Color Fruits

- Lemon, blueberry, raspberry, strawberry watermelon and grapefruit melon. (To be consumed once a week)

- Broccoli

- Brown rice

- Spinach

- Cauliflower

- Cucumber

- Cabbage

- Tomato

- Onion

- Asparagus

- Lean meat and fish

- Lacteous products

- Nuts and seeds

- Olive, coconut and avocado oils

- Spices

Drinks from the keto diet?

- Water

- Coffee

- Tea

- Coconut smoothie

- Bitter chocolate

- Low-carb fruit juices.

Foods to avoid or decrease in the keto diet

- Alcoholic beverages

- Sugared, carbonated or energy drinks

- Bread

- Pasta

- Rice

- Barley

- Oats

- Potatoes

- Candies and sweetmeat.

- Grape, mango, banana, tangerine, apple, date, fig, etc.

- Processed meats

- Wheat flours

- Processed Carbohydrates

- Margarines

- Processed foods

Chapter 7

Can I go on playing Keto forever?

The ketogenic diet is part of a healthy lifestyle and can be perfectly adopted as a permanent eating plan, always taking care of the supply of nutrients that your body needs for its functioning.

A keto diet plan is generally recommended for a period of three months, during which you should see the expected results. However, many people start the ketogenic diet and when they reach their desired weight; they adapt the amounts of macronutrients to their current nutritional needs, continue with the diet and maintain their ideal weight.

In a publication in JAMA magazine, Dr David S. Ludwig, from Haward University, said that a period of adaptation of the body occurs during the diet, and once the diet is stopped; "Hunger increases and metabolism decreases, increasing the tendency to recover fat.

In this sense, it is advisable to adapt the diet to the real nutritional needs of people and maintain this healthy lifestyle

How to avoid the rebound effect, after the diet?

The rebound effect is one of the risks you run when you go on a diet. It is important to maintain eating habits and a healthy lifestyle, to enjoy a state of well-being permanently.

Create healthy habits, such as:

- Eating food in its natural state
- Take control of your life and prepare your meals
- Chew your food well and enjoy its taste.
- Take a nap, without interruptions, after meals.
- Perform the activities of the day at a set time
- Exercise or walk 30 minutes a day
- Sleep 8 hours
- Listen to relaxing music

- Surround yourself with people who want your well-being
- Helping others
- Expresses gratitude
- Read books that nourish your knowledge

The behavior of the kidneys with the Keto diet.

During the ketogenic diet, the kidneys are forced to work excessively, because there is a greater production of urine and elimination of minerals in this process.

Many detractors of the keto diet have been blaming kidney problems on this diet, however, the keto diet is not about eliminating or bringing "zero" carbohydrates and sugars. The minimum percentage of these macro nutrients is 5%, which indicates that this is still an important number and does not have to cause any damage to any organ in the body.

However, there is a greater effort in the work of the kidney during the diet, for this it is important that the person is properly informed of the need to stay hydrated, consume enough water and mineral supplements, and take appropriate precautions for the total success of the diet.

Chapter 8

Tips

- Involve your family group in the importance of the issue of nutrition

- As an empowered team, to which you can delegate functions and reduce stress or burden.

- Increase consumption of fruits and green vegetables.

- Drink broth or consommé 1 or 2 times a day during the first week of the diet.

- Add butter to foods and drinks.

- Add butter to coffee and black chocolate.

- Increase your intake of healthy fats to avoid food cravings or feeling hungry.

- Take vitamin supplements of iron, zinc, calcium, magnesium, among others, making sure they do not contain sugars.

- Cooking techniques; baking, roasting, steaming.

- Green leafy vegetables should be steamed, taking care to maintain their appearance.

- Avoid consumption of cigarettes, drugs and other hallucinogenic substances.

- Read food and medicine labels carefully.

- Avoid using tablets.

- Prefer aspartame and avoid powdered sweeteners.

Conclusion

The keto diet is the most widely used diet worldwide, as a natural dietary treatment in the control of overweight, disease prevention and health improvements. It is now being considered as a powerful weapon against neurogenerative diseases, obesity, diabetes and cardiovascular problems.

For the keto diet to be successful, the family group must be involved, empowered with knowledge for food choice, conservation and preparation.

It is an eating plan that basically recommends the right way to combine macronutrients, to have effects on the body's metabolism.

The keto diet is a strict diet and must be assumed with responsibility, discipline, perseverance and organization, values that ensure its success.

Although there is a false belief that the keto diet implies an investment of large amounts of money, the knowledge about the nutritional value of food and the nutritional needs of your body, are determinants for the correct selection and combination of foods that translate into savings.

Many times people spend unnecessary amounts of money on processed foods that can be replaced by natural ones, which provide greater benefits because they are of high quality and free of toxic substances.

It is important to adopt a healthy lifestyle, forging habits that last over time, maintain balance in the body's biological levels and contribute to improving people's quality of life.

It is an effective diet; the person experiences a feeling of satiety, which guarantees permanent and true results.

The person is not emotionally affected, maintains a good mood and a positive attitude in life, as he or she feels free to choose and enjoy his or her food.

It is a fun and healthy way to live!